TRAVEL PILATES

About the Author

Alida Belair was born in the south of France in 1944, where her parents – Jewish refugees – were in hiding from the Nazis. In 1949 her family emigrated to Melbourne, Australia, where she learnt to dance at the Borovansky Ballet Academy, being declared a 'child prodigy' at a very early age. She was soon selected to dance major roles with a group of Borovansky dancers, taking the ballet from the major cities of Australia to the outback.

At seventeen, Alida became the first Australian to train with the Bolshoi Ballet in Moscow. She went on to become principal ballerina at the famous Ballet Rambert, and then moved to the USA where she was invited to dance leading roles with the National Ballet in Washington, the Chicago Ballet, the New York Ballet, and the prestigious American Ballet Theater.

Alida's relationship with Pilates began in the 1960s and has continued to the present day. She is one of the most sought-after Pilates instructors in Melbourne, where she now lives. Her bestselling autobiography, *Out of Step*, is celebrated as an Australian classic.

TRAVEL PILATES

FITNESS TO GO

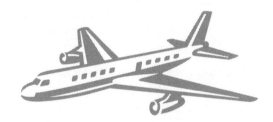

Alida Belair

Published by Schwartz Publishing

Level 5, 289 Flinders Lane
Melbourne Victoria 3000 Australia
email: enquiries@blackincbooks.com
http://www.schwartzpublishing.com

National Library of Australia Cataloguing-in-Publication
entry:

        Belair, Alida, 1944- .
        Travel pilates: fitness to go.
        ISBN 1 86395 269 1.
        1. Pilates method. 2. Stretching exercises.
        3. Physical fitness. I. Title.

        613.71

Photography by Nick Richards
Book design by Thomas Deverall
Printed in Australia by Griffin Press

Contents

Preface

My relationship with Pilates began in the 1960s, when I was a principal ballerina with leading classical ballet companies in Europe and the USA. Like most people who rely on their body for their career, I was struggling to find a balance between the rigors of constant travel and the physical and mental demands of a dancer's life.

Pilates was the answer. With its holistic approach to health and extreme portability, it offered exercises I could adapt to suit almost every environment and situation. When I was in the studio, the attention to alignment and core stability at the heart of the Pilates method was a perfect complement to my ballet regime. And when I was on tour, the breathing technique, stretches and mobilizing exercises were excellent for relieving anxiety and tension.

After I retired, I discontinued Pilates. In my fifties, though, a bad case of 'writer's back' led me to Andrew Baxter's Pilates studio, where I rediscovered the magic of the technique. My transformation was dramatic. Within weeks of resuming Pilates, my head felt clear, my movements became fluid, strong, and controlled, my back pain disappeared, and when I looked in the mirror, it seemed as if I had stepped back into my dancer's body, albeit a slightly more mature one.

When people were generous enough to say how fit I looked, I was able to reassure them that looking toned and healthy at my age, or at any age for that matter, was due not to wishful thinking or to a lucky mix of genes, but rather to the intelligent approach of Pilates. Even more so than when I had been a dancer, I was convinced that the method worked.

My renewed enthusiasm soon inspired me to open my own studio and share the benefits of Pilates with people from all walks of life. The next step followed naturally. Having experienced the benefits of Pilates, many of those I taught felt the need for an easy exercise program for when they were away for an extended period. Trying to keep up a fitness routine while traveling is often inconvenient and impractical at the best of times. Preparing for a journey – rushing to get everything organized at work and at home, making last-minute decisions about what to pack, carrying heavy baggage, dealing with airport delays, ticket hassles, and queues – always takes its toll. A specially designed Pilates-based maintenance program seemed to be the answer. The exercises described in this book, with their focus on the interaction between the brain and body, are specifically designed to help overcome the negative aspects of travel.

*

Scarcely a day goes by without a glowing reference in the media to the benefits of Pilates. Studios and classes are springing up everywhere. What is it about this method – a trade secret with dancers and athletes since the 1930s – that is exciting such a diverse range of people? And given that Joseph Pilates developed his principles in the 1920s, why now?

Perhaps Madonna's well-toned body, and the recommendations of sportspeople such as Tiger Woods and Jason Kidd, partly explain the current burst of popularity. However, I suspect a more substantial factor is the endorsement of the medical profession, which confirms now what Joseph Pilates understood instinctively and formulated through his research all those years ago.

Pilates was fascinated by the healing powers of the mind. He became convinced that it was possible to realign and rebalance the body by altering faulty movement patterns through exercise. He became a passionate advocate for a holistic approach to health and happiness which drew on a wide range of exercise styles and philosophies.

Since Joseph Pilates' groundbreaking ideas were first developed, the method has not remained static. It has evolved and kept pace with new scientific discoveries, new developments in physiology, and new findings about the healthy effect of exercise. Now there are as many interpretations of Pilates as there are teachers.

My own take is an unashamedly hybrid one. In compiling *Travel Pilates* I have drawn on the fundamental principles of Pilates and on a wide range of ideas and methods – from ballet to shiatsu – that have influenced me in my long career as a principal dancer and teacher of Pilates.

Although this book is primarily designed to help Pilates devotees to maintain their physical and mental well-being, I am sure it will also inspire others to discover the benefits of this marvelous method for themselves.

Alida Belair
March 2004

Acknowledgement: I would like to thank Joo-Cheong Tham for appearing in the photographs in this book.

Warning

Travel Pilates is not a substitute for regular sessions with your Pilates instructor, whose role is to assess **your** body and tailor each session to suit **your** specific needs.

Do not attempt any exercises that are beyond your capacity.

You need to be constantly aware of **how** you are exercising. Improperly executed exercises can cause injuries rather than prevent them, so it's important to follow the guidelines carefully.

Pilates is a personal experience. The body is never the same for very long – listen to your body's daily needs and choose, eliminate, and adapt the exercises accordingly. Brilliant as it is, Pilates will not work for you unless you do it regularly.

CAUTION

If you are pregnant or suffer from any illness or injury, always seek medical advice before commencing an exercise routine.

Benefits of Pilates

The thoughtful, low-impact exercises of Pilates challenge the common assumption that exercise needs to be grueling to be effective. They are beneficial at any age or level of fitness.

Pilates works from the inside out, focusing on strengthening the deep postural muscles – this is known as **core stability**.

The Pilates method:

- Heightens body awareness
- Increases lung capacity
- Oxygenates the blood to replenish cells and increase blood flow to the brain
- Reduces stress and fatigue
- Relieves stiffness, pain, and tension
- Strengthens, stretches, and stabilizes
- Prevents injury as core strength develops
- Enables easy and economical movement
- Shapes the body by promoting long, lean muscles

Best of all, Pilates-based exercises are adaptable and minimalist. They can be done almost anywhere, whether it be waiting in a queue or confined in an airplane seat.

Key Principles of Pilates

- Balance
- Breathing
- Centering
- Concentration
- Control
- Flowing movement
- Isolation and integration
- Precision
- Relaxation

THE HUMAN SKELETON

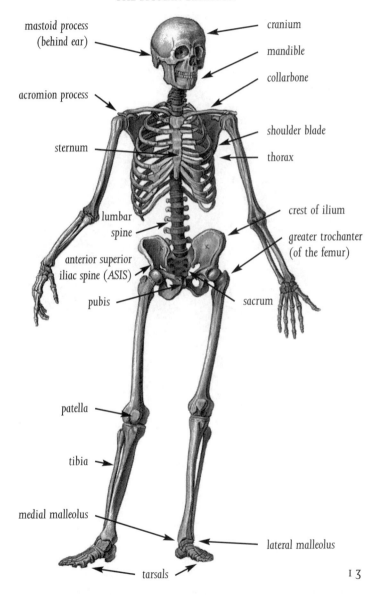

mastoid process (behind ear)

cranium

mandible

collarbone

acromion process

shoulder blade

sternum

thorax

lumbar spine

crest of ilium

anterior superior iliac spine (ASIS)

greater trochanter (of the femur)

pubis

sacrum

patella

tibia

medial malleolus

lateral malleolus

tarsals

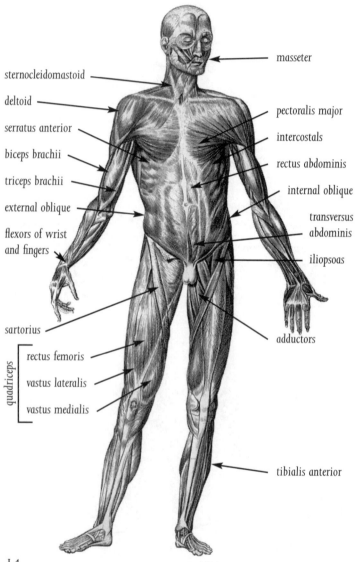

masseter

sternocleidomastoid

deltoid

serratus anterior

biceps brachii

triceps brachii

external oblique

flexors of wrist
and fingers

pectoralis major

intercostals

rectus abdominis

internal oblique

transversus
abdominis

iliopsoas

sartorius

adductors

quadriceps

rectus femoris

vastus lateralis

vastus medialis

tibialis anterior

THE POSTERIOR MUSCLES OF THE BODY

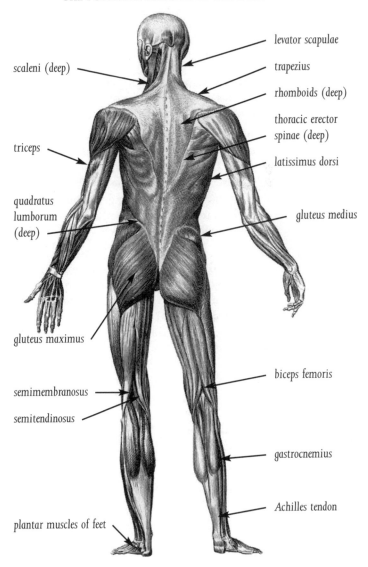

levator scapulae

trapezius

rhomboids (deep)

thoracic erector spinae (deep)

latissimus dorsi

gluteus medius

biceps femoris

gastrocnemius

Achilles tendon

scaleni (deep)

triceps

quadratus lumborum (deep)

gluteus maximus

semimembranosus

semitendinosus

plantar muscles of feet

Pilates: Your Passport to Healthy Travel

Sitting in cramped conditions in a plane, train, car, or bus can have all sorts of nasty effects on your body, and therefore on your mood.

If you are flying, changing time zones will play havoc with your system. The typical symptoms of jet lag are dehydration, indigestion, broken sleep patterns, daytime fatigue, swelling in legs and feet, and a feeling of being in motion for days afterwards. Experts say you need one day per time zone crossed to recover.

In addition, the effect of cabin pressure is similar to that of being high up in the mountains. As the humidity in a cabin is only ten per cent, you may experience the discomforts associated with dehydration and poor air circulation – headaches, sore eyes, and swollen legs and feet. Poor blood circulation may cause Deep Vein Thrombosis (DVT).

But you can easily perform some revitalizing Pilates-based exercises.

Pilates – with its focus on integrating the mind and body – will clear your mind and refresh your body while it corrects the postural imbalances associated with long periods of inactivity.

Breathing – the link between body and mind – is intrinsic to Pilates. It underpins every exercise and ensures that we recruit the deepest support muscles for greater core stability. We need to breathe to live, but not everyone realizes that we need to learn how to breathe correctly.

The conscious breathing in Pilates distributes aerobic muscle food to the body and brain. Then, as we use all of our lung capacity, our energy lifts and our concentration and mental functioning improve.

If you are not relaxed, your breathing will be affected.

First, it helps to settle down in your seat and check your posture. This can be done even before the plane takes off. Then a breathing exercise will replenish body and mind.

Set your watch to the time at your destination so you can plan onboard naps.

Coffee and tea are dehydrating and the effects of alcohol are doubled. Drink about eight ounces of water for every hour of flight.

Avoid eating fatty, rich foods and snacking out of boredom.

On the Way

De-Stress, Tone, Stretch, Relax

CONTROLLED BREATHING

To alleviate stress and anxiety, keep the blood flowing, and prevent ankles from swelling

Sit as upright as you can, heels together and pressing against the mat. Feel the trunk lift and lengthen away from the pelvic girdle.

Inhale through the nose for 3 counts.

Exhale through the mouth for 3 counts.

[6 reps attaining a gentle rhythm]

If you are very anxious and your breath has become shallow, visualize your lungs slowly filling with air like a balloon when you inhale and deflating as you exhale.

Inhale for 3 counts. Expand the ribcage laterally.

Exhale for 4 counts. The diaphragm relaxes; the ribcage moves down closer toward the pelvis.

[6 reps]

Inhale for 3 counts.

Exhale for 6 counts.

[6 reps]

Watchpoints

Pull up to sit taller on each exhalation. On each repetition, press feet down on the exhalation so that you set up a rhythm.

Inhale for 3 counts.

Exhale for 3 counts. Push down through feet.

[6 reps]

Now inhale for 3 counts and exhale for 6 counts. Continue to inhale for 3 counts and exhale for 6 counts.

[10 reps]

CALMING EXERCISE

To calm the nerves, increase lung capacity, free up the neck, open up the chest, and stretch the upper to mid-back

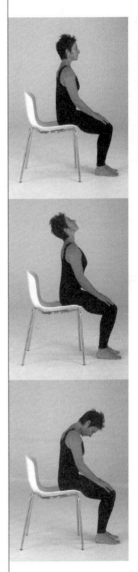

Sit tall on your sitting bones, feet together, heels down.

Inhale. Lift your chin and look upward. Take your upper back into extension.

Exhale. Drop your head down gently. Take your upper back into flexion.

Keep your lower back upright.

Inhale.

Exhale. Come back upright, stacking the vertebrae back on top of each other, bone by bone.

[6 reps]

The Pelvic Floor

The guiding principle of the Pilates technique is that all energy emanates from our center – encompassing the abdominals, hips, buttocks, lower back, and pelvic floor. Joseph Pilates called this the **Powerhouse**.

Most people, particularly men, hardly know that their pelvic floor exists, let alone that it needs to be exercised just like any other muscle group.

A well-toned pelvic floor is not only essential to structural fitness, but also a key ingredient for overall well-being. The pelvic floor cradles the organs in the abdomen, flattens the stomach, and increases sexual satisfaction. These muscles are also linked to the respiratory diaphragm and, therefore, any tension in this area inhibits breathing, as well as movement and speech.

Practice your pelvic lifts en route – while you are staving off boredom, you are strengthening one of the most important structures of the body.

PELVIC FLOOR LIFT 1

To develop an awareness of the link between the diaphragm and the pelvic floor, increase pelvic stabilization, and tone the muscles of the pelvic floor

Sit tall on your chair with your feet planted on the mat.

Inhale. Push down on both feet with equal pressure, relax abdominals and pelvic floor muscles.

Exhale. Lift muscles between tailbone and pubic bone. As your breath runs out, contract higher up the abdomen and feel your transversus abdominis pull across and inward. Keep squeezing the air out and lifting the pelvic floor. Release and let the pelvic floor lower.

The duration of the exhalation should be 6 seconds, with a short inhalation between each rep.

[4 reps]

PELVIC FLOOR LIFT 2

As for Pelvic Floor Lift 1, plus to lengthen the base of the spine, and develop an awareness of correct alignment

Sit tall on your chair.

Place index finger of right hand on your tailbone and place your left hand on the lower abdominals.

Inhale.

Exhale for 6 seconds and lift the pelvic floor a few times.

Inhale. Push down on feet.

Exhale. Close your eyes and visualize that you are stopping your urine mid-flow. Hold, let go – hold longer, let go, hold longer and so on.

Inhale. Release pelvic floor and relax with a sigh.

This exercise can also be done standing with feet parallel and slightly bent knees.

or

While walking, lift the pelvic floor as you take a step and relax it as your foot comes down. Build up to lifting the pelvic floor for several steps.

PELVIC FLOOR LIFT 3

Inhale.

Exhale. Lift the pelvic floor.

Hold.

Inhale. Continue to hold muscles.

Exhale. Lift pelvic floor higher.

Inhale. Hold.

Exhale. Lower pelvic floor a little.

Inhale. Hold.

Exhale. Lower pelvic floor right down.

Inhale. Release pelvic floor and relax with a sigh.

[4 Reps]

Watchpoint

Do not overdo these exercises, as the pelvic floor muscles tire easily and can become overly tense.

Countering the ill-effects of immobility

When you are seated in a confined space for any length of time, your hip muscles will contract and stiffen.

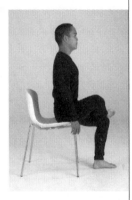

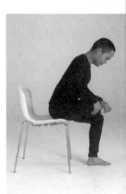

SEATED HIP STRETCH

To mobilize the hip muscles and encourage blood flow

Sit on your chair with your back supported and your feet planted on the mat.

Feel a direct line from midway through the pelvic floor to the crown of your head. Your head should float on a continuum with the spine — neither jolting forward nor pulled back. Relax your shoulders and neck.

Inhale. Slide right foot along left shin and place on left knee.

Exhale. Lean forward to increase stretch on right hip.

Inhale. Hold.

Exhale, long and slow.

Inhale, curving forward as far as possible.

Exhale.

Inhale.

Exhale. Bring your body back to upright position.

Alternate legs.

[2 reps each side]

SHOULDER ROTATIONS

To mobilize the shoulders and relieve tension in the neck and shoulders

Sit tall, place your hands on your shoulders and keep your elbows out to the side.

Inhale. Circle your arms forward and try to get the elbows to touch.

Exhale. Lift your elbows up towards your ears and circle elbows back as far as you can. Isolate the movement to the shoulder area.

Complete the circle, then reverse cycle: back, up, around, and down.

Careful! Don't tense the neck and shoulder muscles or jut the chin forward.

[10 reps in each direction]

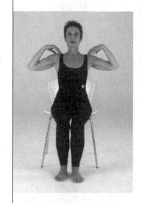

Watchpoint

Carrying heavy bags strains the area between the neck and shoulder. These stretching exercises help relieve stiffness and correct postural bad habits such as raising shoulders, poking the neck and chin forward, rounding the shoulders, and hanging the head.

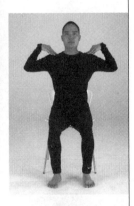

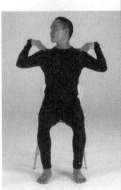

HEAD SWIVELS
To free up the head, neck, and shoulders

Sit upright on your sitting bones, feet together and heels flat on the mat.

Inhale. Place your fingertips on the tops of both shoulders. Direct your elbows sideways. Press down on your tailbone.

Exhale. Lift pelvic floor and pull in abdominis transversus while turning your head toward your left shoulder.

Inhale. Return your head back to the center.

Exhale. Turn your head toward your right shoulder.

Inhale. Return your head back to the center.

Exhale. Relax.

[4 reps]

SHOULDER STRETCH

Sit in your seat with your feet evenly balanced on the mat. Recruit your abdominals and drop your tailbone.

Inhale. Lift your right arm up toward the ceiling.

Exhale. Place your hand on your left shoulder blade, palm facing away.

Inhale. Slide your left hand, palm facing away, up your back. Try to clasp your other hand.

Don't worry if your hands don't touch.

Exhale. Hold the stretch, breathing normally for about 20 seconds. Keep your elbows vertical.

Inhale. Return arms to your side.

Exhale. Relax.

Alternate sides.

[2 reps each side]

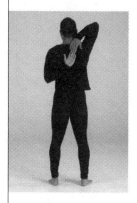

This can be done standing with your legs parallel and hip-width apart.

NECK STRETCH

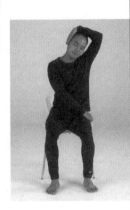

Sit facing straight ahead, feet comfortably apart, heels on the mat.

Inhale. Hold onto the seatbelt or your left hip with your right hand.

Drop your chin diagonally toward your left knee, keeping your right shoulder square with the left shoulder.

Exhale. Place your left palm on the right side of your head, drop your head forward and to the left, keeping your trunk upright.

Hold for 20 seconds.

Breathe in and out.

You should feel a comfortable stretch, not a painful pull.

Relax and alternate.

[2 reps each side]

Upper Body Stretch 1

This stretch lengthens the sides as well as strengthening the shoulders and arms, particularly the triceps

Sit on your seat, feet parallel and pressed on the mat. Interlace your fingers on your lap.

Recruit abdominals, keep a neutral spine.

Inhale.

Exhale. Push your palms toward the ceiling. Try to straighten your arms. Slide your shoulder blades down your back at the same time. Pull outer edges of arms forwards as you push up through your palms.

Inhale.

Exhale. Lower your hands back onto your lap.

[4 reps]

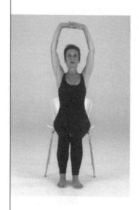

Watchpoints

Keep lumbar spine supported by recruiting abdominals.

Keep your neck and head free of tension.

Feel as if you are lengthening the spine.

UPPER BODY STRETCH 2

To mobilize and strengthen shoulder blades, stretch chest muscles, relieve tension, and re-align neck, shoulders, and spine

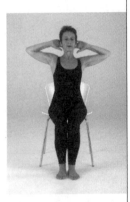

Sit with feet planted on the mat, back upright. Raise hands to chest level and touch your finger tips together, palms facing.

Inhale. Raise your arms, keeping your fingers connected and place them against the back of the hollow of the neck.

Exhale. Feel your shoulder blades slide together and hold your elbows to the side.

Inhale. Lower your head forward.

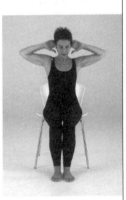

Exhale. Lift your head, lengthen neck, press head against hands. Keep your eyes focused on the front.

Inhale. Bring your hands back onto your thighs.

Exhale.

[3 reps]

Upper Body Stretch 3

To strengthen and re-align neck and upper back

Sit upright on your chair, hands on your thighs, feet parallel on the mat.

Check that your shoulders are down, with your shoulder blades in their stabilized position (pulled down your back into a V shape).

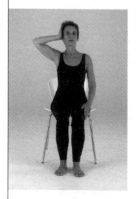

Inhale. Press the fingers of your right hand together and hold the right side of your head just above your ear. Your elbow should be directed to the side.

Exhale. Press your head against your hand for 6 counts.

Lengthen your spine by imagining that you have a string attached from the crown of your head to the ceiling.

Lower your hand back to your thigh.

[4 reps with your right hand]

[4 reps with your left hand]

Upper Body Stretch 4

To restore the balance between the muscle groups of the upper back and to strengthen and stretch the front and back muscles of the upper body

This exercise can be done wherever there is some wall space and could be done while you are waiting to use the toilet.

Stand facing the wall, approximately 18 inches (45 cm) away.

Stretch your arms out sideways at about shoulder height, press hands against the wall. Bend your knees.

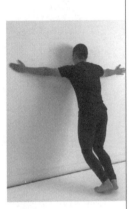

Inhale. Press your feet into the mat.

Exhale. Lean into the wall and bend your elbows. You can slightly lift your heels. Hinge your trunk in line with your toes and ankles toward the wall then slowly push against the wall.

Hold for 6 counts.

Come back to the start and relax.

[5 reps]

Stretch for Calves & Hips

To stretch muscles and to keep the blood circulating (to prevent DVT)

Stand and put your hands on the wall at shoulder height and shoulder width apart, with fingers pointed up to the ceiling.

Take a large step backwards. Keep your heels together and press them down into the mat. The further back you stand the more intense the stretch will be.

Inhale.

Exhale. Raise your left knee and press it towards the wall, keeping the right heel on the mat.

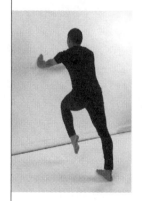

> Ensure that your abdominals are engaged to fully support your lumbar spine. There should be a straight line running from the center of your head to the back of your heel.

Inhale. Bring your leg down next to the other.

Exhale. Raise your right knee and press it toward the wall.

Inhale. Put your right leg down next to the left.

Exhale to finish.

Alternate legs.

[10 reps each side]

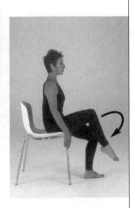

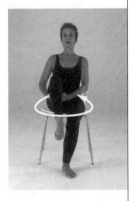

FOOT CIRCLES

To mobilize the feet and ankles and to keep the blood circulating (to prevent DVT)

Sit tall – heels together, feet flat on mat.

Inhale. Lift your right leg.

Exhale. Circle your foot upwards in clockwise direction with pointed foot.

[10 reps]

[10 reps anticlockwise]

Repeat with other leg.

KNEE CIRCLES

To mobilize the knee and promote blood flow

Inhale. Lift your right knee, placing hands under your thigh to support the weight of the leg.

Exhale. Flex your foot and circle your leg at the knee.

[10 reps]

Reverse direction.

[10 reps]

Alternate legs.

[10 reps for each cycle]

CAUTION

Avoid this exercise if you are currently having knee problems.

These rotations should be done as often as possible during the trip.

FOOT MASSAGE

To develop sensitivity, strengthen the intrinsic muscles of the feet, take blood to the feet, and restore mobility

To be done in socks or stockings.

Sit upright on sitting bones, heels together, flat on mat.

Lift your right leg.

Inhale. Place your toes down onto the mat. Roll through onto the ball of your foot.

Exhale. Stroke whole foot along mat until it is beside the other foot.

Begin again.

[10 reps with left foot]

[10 reps with right foot]

TRACKING KNEE

To re-align the leg by focusing on moving the kneecap correctly, to strengthen the knee and to keep blood circulating in the legs (to prevent DVT)

Sit upright on your sitting bones with legs parallel, heels pressing into the mat. If you have something handy like a small pillow, place it between your knees.

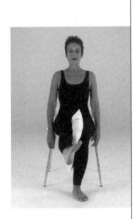

Inhale.

Exhale. Raise right leg, straighten knee, flex foot and turn it inwards. Be careful to isolate the ankle. Place your fingers against the inside muscles above the knee and feel them contract.

Hold for 6 seconds.

[10 reps with right leg]

[10 reps with left leg]

QUADRICEPS STRETCH
To stretch the front thigh muscles

These muscles will tighten considerably when you are sitting for extended periods.

Hold onto something stable, like the back of a seat or side of a car, with your right hand.

Reach behind you with your left hand and take hold of left foot. Keep your knees in line with one another.

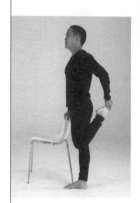

Pull your foot up behind you.

Engage your abdominals and keep your pelvis stable and in neutral.

Keep your hip bones level and on the same plane as your pubic bone.

Hold for 20 seconds, incorporating the Pilates breathing technique.

Alternate legs.

[2 reps each side]

PECTORALS STRETCH
To open up the chest and enhance the breathing

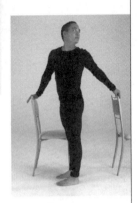

Stand up next to your seat, facing the back.

Hold onto the back of your seat with your right hand and place your left hand on the back of the seat in front of you.

Inhale.

Exhale. Rotate your body away from your right hand towards the seat.

Alternate.

[2 reps each side]

Hip & Lower Back Stretch

To massage the internal organs

> This stretch aids digestion; long trips can cause constipation.

Stand next to your seat in the aisle.

Inhale. Slowly and carefully slide your right foot up your left leg until you can take hold of your right knee with both hands. (If necessary, steady yourself by holding onto the seat with one hand.)

Exhale. Pull the knee upwards towards your trunk.

Inhale.

Exhale. Slide your foot back down beside the other.

Alternate legs.

[10 reps each side]

Watchpoints

Keep abdominals recruited.

Lengthen spine. Imagine that there is a string attached to the crown of your head at one end and to the ceiling at the other.

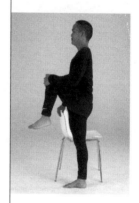

Massage

Mental tension is often expressed in stiffness of the body, particularly in the upper body.

Self-massage can be a surprisingly effective way of relieving tension. It helps restore balance to the body by equalizing muscle tone on both sides as well as stimulating blood circulation.

A former ballet teacher of mine taught me these simple Jin Shin Jyutsu exercises to help beat jet lag. Once again, the great thing about these simple little exercises is that you can do them anywhere.

MASSAGE EXERCISE 1

Hold the thumb of your left hand with the fingers of your right and focus on what you are doing. When you can feel a steady pulse, move on, working your way through all the fingers of your left hand.

Repeat the exercise on the right hand.

MASSAGE EXERCISE 2

1 Interlace your fingers and rub your palms together. Release, then move one space along and massage your palms again.

2 Make fists with your hands and then release. Make fists again and circle your wrists 10 times clockwise and 10 times anticlockwise.

3 Put the fingertips of your right hand on your left shoulder and massage with circular motions along the top of your shoulder blade.

4 Move down to the collarbone and massage down your upper arm.

5 Move your hand up the side of your neck to the top of your head and massage firmly, turning your head left and right slowly at the same time.

6 Place your left hand just below the collarbone on your right side and gently massage your chest.

7 Place your left hand just below your right armpit. If the muscles beneath your ribs feel tight, your shoulder blades will stiffen. Massage with firm circular movements.

8 Now massage gently along and across the ribs with your left hand.

9 Finally, move back up the side of your neck to the top of your head and massage firmly.

Repeat from step 3, swapping arm.

SOOTHE EYE STRAIN

The recycled air and dryness in a plane can make you feel lethargic, bring on headaches, block your ears, and affect your eyes.

As well as using saline drops to replenish the moisture in your eyes, you can do these simple exercises:

1 Cup your hands over your eyes, keeping them open.

2 Press your fingers to the spot just above your eyebrows and pause for 20 seconds.

3 Move your fingers to the hollows at the side of your nose just beside your eyes – hold for 20 seconds.

4 Pull gently down your nose from the top to the end.

5 Press under your cheekbones for 20 seconds.

6 Place the cups of your hands back over your eyes, keeping them open.

WALKING AS MEDITATION

In order to counter DVT it is important to keep your muscles moving. Walk down the aisle from time to time. Focus on your steps.

Feel your feet touch the mat. How does the mat feel? Be aware of your five toes spreading as you walk. Can you feel the foot move from heel to toe?

Focus on breathing.

Firstly, inhale to lift the foot.

Now exhale to take a step.

Do this for a while then switch to taking three steps on the inhalation and then three steps on the exhalation.

Relaxation Exercise

If you are in an airplane, lower your food tray.

If you are in a bus, car, or plane you may use your soft hand luggage or a pillow for support.

Allow your whole upper body to rest fully supported on the tray.

Put your forehead on your hands and focus on relaxing.

Concentrate on breathing with a slow easy rhythm.

Inhale for 6 seconds.

Exhale for 6 seconds.

> *Feel your rib cage expand on the inhalations and deflate on the exhalations.*

[5 reps, or more]

When You're There

Warm Up, Workout, Wind Down

Your daily workout

You will need

Floor space: enough to lie down full-length

Wall space: approximately 7 feet (2 meters)

Blanket or exercise mat to lie on

Towel and/or Thera-Band

Small pillow

Chair

Clothes that allow free movement

15 minutes, $1/2$ hour or 1 hour, 3–4 times per week

The exercises in this chapter will help you put together your own workout, depending on how much time you have and how you feel. It's best to stick to the exercises that you already know and those that you can do safely without an instructor.

Pilates exercises are formulated to be muscle-specific. However, while you are overtly working your shoulder rotators or leg adductors, your trunk stabilizers should kick in simultaneously. So you will often experience muscle engagement in several parts of the body at the same time.

It is important to balance your workout. Pilates exercises fall into three general categories that often overlap:

- Strengthening
- Mobility
- Flexibility

If the level of the exercises is advanced, this is indicated with an *A.

Never rush. The most important things are control and precision. If you are strapped for time, limit the number of exercises and go for quality rather than quantity.

Focus on your alignment and then on each movement, making sure that you are targeting the correct group of muscles.

Modify your program to suit your daily needs. For example, when you have had a particularly hectic schedule, you may want to incorporate more stretches and reduce the number of strengthening exercises.

Your workout can be done anytime, although it is wise not to exercise immediately after eating. Work at your own pace and stop if anything hurts.

All people are structurally different, learn at different speeds, and work at different tempos. Although I have devised three sample programs – long, medium, and short – these are only a guide.

Always prepare your body for exercise by warming up before you begin.

Pilates must be holistic to be effective – try not to favor the exercises you enjoy or come most easily to you.

THE ESSENTIAL PRINCIPLES
- CONCENTRATION
- BREATHING
- ISOLATION
- INTEGRATION
- PRECISION
- CONTROL
- CENTERING
- FLOWING MOVEMENT
- RELAXATION

Stretching & Warming Up

You need to warm up to release fluids into your joints. Otherwise, your muscles will not be pliable and the risk of injury will increase.

These stretches can be incorporated into your workout at the beginning to warm up or at the end to wind down. Listen to your body – it will tell you which stretches will suit your daily needs.

FULL BODY STRETCH
To integrate body and mind and stimulate blood circulation

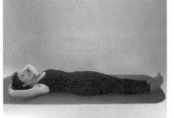

Lie on your back. Clasp your hands at the crown of your head. Bend your elbows. Relax your feet.

Inhale.

Exhale. Stretch arms behind you. Take your shoulders into a shrug (abduction). Flex your feet.

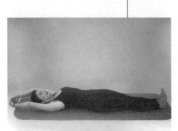

Inhale. Bend your elbows. Bring shoulders back to neutral, return hands to the crown of the head.

Exhale. Relax feet.

[10 reps]

ARM OPENING

To promote a sense of openness across the chest, stabilize the spine, and rotate the spine

Lie on your side with your head on a rolled towel.

Bend your knees at a right angle. Line your back up in neutral. Extend your arms at shoulder height with your palms together.

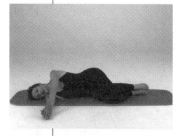

Inhale. Lift upper arm.

Exhale. Keep elbow soft and open to the side. Follow your hand with your eyes so that your head follows the direction of the arm as it moves. Try to touch the mat with your arm (don't force it). Keep knees together and abdominals recruited – hollowing to the backbone.

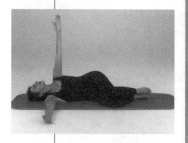

Inhale and exhale slowly while holding the chest in its open position.

Inhale. Bring your arm back in an arc overhead, eyes following.

Exhale as you return your hand to rest, palm on palm.

[5 reps each side]

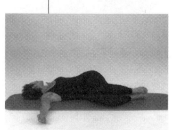

BASIC WALL STRETCH I

To improve the blood circulation in your legs and feet

Imperative if you have been sitting still or standing for any length of time.

Sit sideways. Get your buttocks close up to the wall.

Roll on to your back. Place your legs on the wall in parallel, hip-width apart. Keep your tailbone on the mat and your back in neutral. If your hamstrings are tight, move a little further from the wall and bend your knees. Relax your arms beside you. Keep your shoulder blades pulled down. Your neck should feel free and relaxed.

Circle feet outwards.

[10 reps]

Circle feet inwards.

[10 reps]

Work feet at the ankles and keep legs parallel.

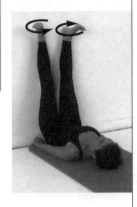

BASIC WALL STRETCH II
To stretch hamstrings and front of legs

Position same as Basic Wall Stretch I, keeping your legs parallel.

Point and flex.

[10 reps]

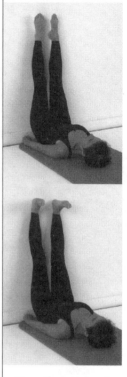

The calf muscles work more intensely when the legs are elevated.

When the leg muscles are contracted and released, they assist the return of blood to the heart.

In addition, these exercises relax and expand the upper body.

53

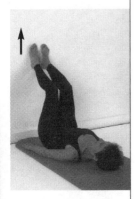

EXERCISE FOR TIRED FEET

Keep wall position.

Move away from the wall a little. Bend your knees, keeping feet flat on the wall.

Spread your toes, then scrunch them as if you are going to pick up a pencil. Your feet will creep up the wall a little.

Keep scrunching and creeping your feet until they cannot remain flat.

INNER THIGH MUSCLE STRETCH

Keep your wall position.

Rest your legs straight up the wall, either parallel or turned out.

Slowly widen your legs to the side. Keep your feet against the wall.

Once you have arrived at your maximum stretch, stay there for 30 seconds. Breathe using your Pilates technique.

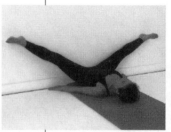

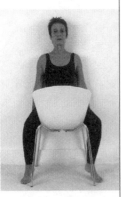

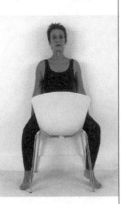

SHOULDER SHRUGS WITH WEIGHTS

To reduce tension in shoulders and neck

You'll need 2 x 1.25-liter bottles of soft drink or similar weighted objects.

Straddle a chair with your back facing a wall.

Your shoulder blades and pelvis should be supported by the wall. Your feet should be flat on the mat if possible. Let your arms dangle vertically from your shoulders and hold a weight in each hand.

Inhale. Shrug your shoulders up towards your ears and hold this position for 5 seconds.

Exhale. Let your shoulder blades slide down the wall as your shoulders lower.

[20 reps]

SIDE STRETCH

Straddle a chair.

Hold on to the left side of the back of the chair. Keep your shoulders square. Hang your right arm vertically by your side. Keep your feet flat on the mat if possible.

Inhale. Lengthen through the spine and raise your right arm over your head.

Exhale. Reach over to the left side.

Imagine that you are trying to touch the opposite wall with your right hand. Keep the spine elongated and think of lengthening horizontally rather than crunching down towards the mat.

Inhale. Return to upright position with your arm over your head.

Exhale. Bring your right arm down and repeat with the other arm.

[6 reps each side]

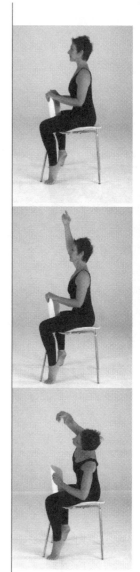

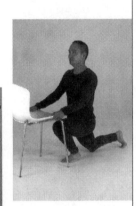

HIP FLEXOR STRETCH
To stretch the quadriceps and iliopsoas

Take a lunge position, holding onto a chair to balance. Keep your knee vertical to your ankle.

Inhale. Kneel on the other leg, foot behind you.

Recruit the abdominals.

Exhale. Press hips forward. Feel the stretch.

If you feel confident, take your hands off the chair and rest them on your knee.

Alternate.

[2 reps each side]

Calf Stretch

Stand approximately 18" (45 cm) away from the wall, facing it. Legs straight, feet together.

Place your hands against the wall.

Inhale. Bend your knees, lift right foot, and press lifted toes against the wall.

Exhale. Stretch your calf gently by straightening front leg.

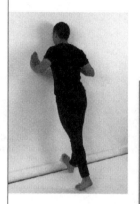

Move both hips forward by pushing on the ball of the back foot. The heel will come off the mat.

Hold for 6 seconds.

Do not bounce or force the stretch.

Alternate legs.

[2 reps each side]

Supine Hamstring Stretch
To improve hamstring flexibility

You'll need a towel or Thera-Band.

Lie on your back. Bend knees (constructive rest).

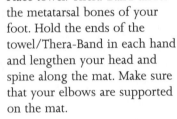

Raise one leg with bent knee.

Place towel/Thera-Band under the metatarsal bones of your foot. Hold the ends of the towel/Thera-Band in each hand and lengthen your head and spine along the mat. Make sure that your elbows are supported on the mat.

Inhale. Stretch your knee and lengthen your leg diagonally away from the center of your body.

Exhale. If you have enough flexibility, stretch your other leg down the mat. If not, leave the knee bent.

Inhale.

Exhale. Draw your extended leg up towards a 90-degree angle. Make sure your buttock remains pressed on the mat as you lengthen your heel up to the ceiling.

Inhale.

Exhale. Try to release further into the stretch.

Repeat for 3 further breaths, gently easing into the stretch on each exhalation.

Inhale. Bend the knee back.

Exhale. Lower the leg to the mat, stretching it out alongside the other leg.

Alternate legs.

[2 reps each side]

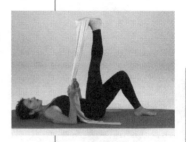

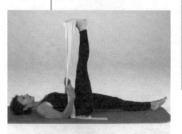

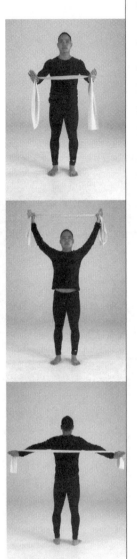

CHEST STRETCH
To mobilize rotator muscles in the shoulders and open the chest

You can use either a towel or a Thera-Band.

Stand with your feet parallel, hip-width apart. Hold the towel/Thera-Band with both hands, approximately 18" (45 cm) apart or slightly wider than your shoulders. Make sure that your shoulder blades are stabilized. Hold towel/Thera-Band in front of you, elbows soft.

Inhale. Bring your hands up over your head. Contract your abdominals. Keep the shoulders drawn down your back. Take particular care not to project the ribs forward. Don't lose the connection between the ribcage and the backbone.

Exhale. Continue the movement. Take your arms over your head, holding arms straight. Now take the arms behind you as far as you can, allowing the hands to move further apart.

Inhale. Bring the arms back overhead.

Exhale. Bring the arms forward to the starting position.

[10 reps]

Turtle

To mobilize the shoulder blades, stabilize the shoulder girdle, and work deep neck flexors

This exercise releases tension in the neck.

Lie prone with your feet together and your forehead on the mat.

Place your arms wide apart so that your shoulder blades are not pinching together, elbows are bent at right angles, and hands are resting on the mat.

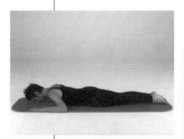

Inhale.

Exhale. Contract abdominals to spine, press down into the arms, bring up head and chest. Keep elbows on the mat as your neck extends out of the shoulder girdle away from the base of the spine. Keep your head floating on a continuum with your spine. Pull your shoulder blades down into a V shape. Try to relax the buttocks and use only upper to mid-back.

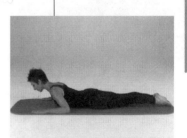

Inhale. Lower your head to the mat and let your shoulders relax and your spine resettle.

[10 reps]

SINGLE & DOUBLE LEG & ARM STRETCH (SWIMMING)

To develop core strength, with the focus on centering and lengthening. Strengthens abdominals, glutei, and erector spinae

Single Leg Stretch

Lie prone.

You may want to roll a towel and place it under your forehead, to keep your head in line with your neutral spine. Stretch arms overhead (lengthening) and point feet in opposite direction (also lengthening).

Inhale.

Exhale. Draw in abdominals.

> *Imagine that there is something sharp on the mat and that you are lifting away from it. This is the support for your lumbar spine.*

Lift arm and opposite leg.

> *Do not lift too high — think of lengthening and releasing the limbs from the joints, rather than lifting. Keep both hips on mat. Do not twist the torso or limbs. Your head should be slightly higher than the parallel of your arm.*

Inhale. Lower limbs and relax.

Alternate sides.

[10 reps each side]

Exhale. Relax.

Double Arm & Leg Stretch

Lie prone, as in Single Leg Stretch.

Inhale.

Exhale. Lift both arms and legs.

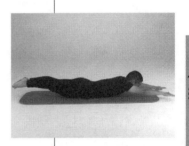

Stretch away from your center in opposite directions. Think of stretching and releasing, rather than lifting.

Inhale. Lower limbs to mat and relax.

[10 reps]

Exhale. Relax.

SERGEANT MAJOR (THE DART)

To strengthen the shoulder girdle and back and to develop core stability

A great warm-up exercise.

Lie prone, arms by your sides. Keep legs straight and in line with your head and spine.

Inhale.

Exhale. Slide shoulder blades down your back. Lift head and feet off the mat.

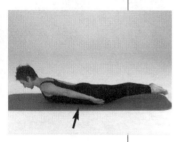

Be careful to engage your pelvic floor and abdominals in order to protect the lumbar spine.

Stretch arms down your thighs, pulling your hands towards your feet.

Don't come up too high with your head — it should look as if you are standing to attention.

Inhale. Lower down and release.

Focus on lengthening from your toes to the crown of your head and visualize the transversus abdomini supporting the back underneath.

[10 reps]

Exhale. Relax.

THE CAT

To undulate the spine and integrate the upper and lower spine

Position yourself on all fours with your back in neutral, hands directly under shoulders, knees directly under hips. Your head should float on a continuum with your spine.

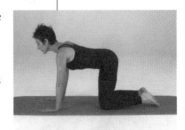

Inhale.

Exhale. Contract abdominals, pulling them up into your backbone. Take your spine into flexion, remembering to keep your head in alignment with the curve.

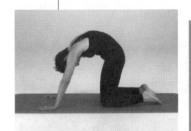

Inhale. Take your spine back to neutral.

Exhale. Take your spine into extension. Bring the head up in line with the curve.

Inhale. Take your spine back to neutral.

[10 reps]

Exhale. Relax.

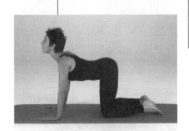

PELVIC ROCK
To articulate the base of the spine

Lie on your back, knees in constructive rest (this may be done with a small pillow between your knees).

Inhale.

Exhale. Lift your tailbone off the mat.

Inhale. Lower tailbone back onto the mat and lengthen your spine.

Use a gentle rhythmic rocking motion.

[10 reps]

Exhale. Relax.

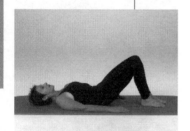

PELVIC PRESS

To mobilize spine, increase the flexibility of the lower back, coordinate muscles of legs and pelvis, and challenge the abdominals

This exercise may be done with a pillow between the knees.

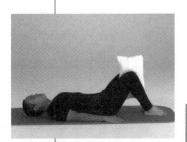

Lie on your back, legs in constructive rest, feet flat and parallel, arms by your side. Slide shoulder blades down your spine and lengthen your arms away. Rest head on mat (no pillow).

Inhale.

Exhale. Slowly peel the spine off the mat, one bone at a time, raising hips towards the ceiling to form a bridge.

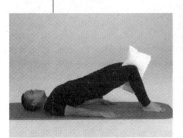

Inhale. Keep your form.

Exhale. Lower spine, one bone at a time, beginning from the top of the thoracic spine and continuing until the tailbone comes back to rest on the mat.

> *Make the movements slow and fluent. Make sure that when your spine is raised, your knees, hips, and back are aligned with the shoulders, and your neck and head are in line with your spine. Keep head, neck, and shoulders flat on the mat throughout.*

[10 reps]

Abdominal Preparation

To isolate and recruit the pelvic floor and abdominals, work inside thigh muscles, and expand lower back (great for sciatica sufferers)

Lie on your back, with knees in constructive rest. Place a pillow between your knees. You may want to place a rolled towel under your head. Spine should be neutral, arms by your side. Place hands at the back of your head just behind your ears, keeping elbows directed to the side.

Inhale. Raise your head and shoulders, using the xiphoid process as a fulcrum.

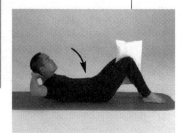

Keep your ribs anchored to the mat. Gaze at the tops of your knees.

Exhale. Zip up the muscles of the pelvic floor and scoop your abdominals to your backbone. Squeeze the pillow between your knees. Do not tuck pelvis or lift tailbone.

Inhale. Roll back down to the mat, bone by bone. Release your knees.

Exhale. Let spine resettle along the mat.

[10 reps]

ABDOMINAL CURL
To strengthen abdominals

Lie on your back, with knees in constructive rest. You may want to place a
rolled towel or small pillow under your
head and a pillow between your knees.

Spine neutral – hands behind head, as
in Abdominal Preparation.

Inhale. Lengthen your spine.

Exhale. Raise head and shoulders. Keep
neck lengthened and chin dropped
slightly (not over-retracted). Contract
abdominals, but remain anchored in
the middle of the pelvis.

You should aim for a lengthened curve
with the transversus and the oblique
muscles controlling the rectus abdominus.

Inhale. Release abdominals by 10 per
cent.

Exhale. Contract abdominals again.

[10 reps]

Then inhale and roll your spine down
to the mat, bone by bone.

Exhale. Relax.

Tip

*So as not to strain your
neck, imagine holding
a tennis ball under
your chin during this
exercise.*

ROLL UP 1 *A

This is an alternative to the Abdominal Preparation and the Abdominal Curl.

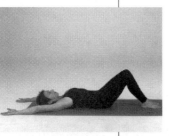

Lie supine, legs in constructive rest, arms behind head, spine lengthened.

Inhale. Raise your arms overhead and then bring them down towards your legs.

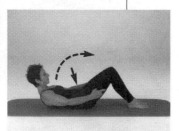

Roll your head and shoulders bone by bone up to the shoulder blades at the back. Use the xiphoid process as the fulcrum in the front.

Exhale. Continue to pluck the bones off one by one until you are sitting upright with your legs straight out in front of you. Keep heels together and parallel.

Inhale. Raise your arms over-head to lengthen the spine.

Exhale. With three pulses, stretch arms and back over legs towards your flexed feet. This stretches the back and hamstrings.

Inhale. Begin to roll down, bone by bone. Lead with your tail-bone, sacrum, and lumbar, taking your arms overhead.

Keep scooping, draw your knees up.

Exhale and continue to roll until you are lying back on the mat in your constructive rest position.

[10 reps]

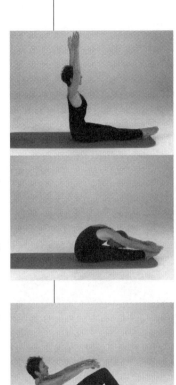

Roll Up ii *A

Once you have mastered Roll Up i, try the more advanced version.

Begin as at left, keeping your legs straight.

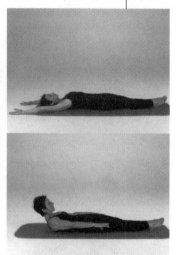

Inhale. Raise your arms overhead and lower them until they are next to your thighs. Bring head and shoulders off the mat. Use the xiphoid process as the fulcrum.

Exhale. Slowly roll off the mat, bone by bone.

Continue to roll forward until you can place your hands on the balls of your feet to emphasize the hamstring stretch.

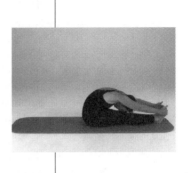

Inhale. Remain in the stretch.

Exhale. Roll back down to the mat – bone by bone, leading with the tailbone, sacrum, etc.

[10 reps]

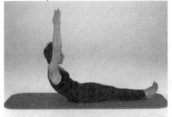

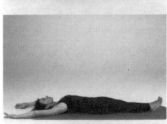

SPINE ROLL-UP *A

To articulate the spine, strengthen the abdominals, and promote fluidity

CAUTION

If you have an injury such as a bad neck or back, give the roll-up a miss.

The roll-up relies on maximum use of the powerhouse and should not be attempted by anyone who is unfamiliar with this exercise.

Lie flat on the mat with neutral spine, stretched legs, pointed feet, and ankles and thighs held together.

Rest arms by your sides, palms down.

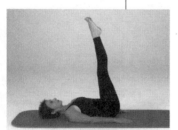

Inhale. Lift legs to 90 degrees.

Exhale. Move legs towards your head and begin to peel your bones off the mat, bone by bone, beginning with the tailbone.

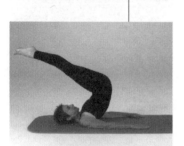

Imagine that you are trying to attach your tailbone to the ceiling. Your spine is lengthening upwards, defying gravity. Control the roll-up with your powerhouse.

Don't worry if your legs are not parallel to the ceiling and mat. It is more important to focus on lengthening through the spine and lifting through the hips. Your abdominals form the inside support wall of your pose.

Do not roll legs overhead and let the spine collapse. Your weight should be supported across your shoulder blades, not by your neck.

Inhale. Open legs to shoulder width. Flex feet. Imagine that you have lead weights in your feet.

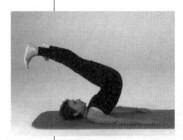

Exhale. Begin to roll back, bone by bone, onto the mat, beginning with the upper spine. Use your straight legs and feet as counter-weights and control the wheeling with your power-house.

When your tailbone has touched down and resettled, lower your legs to about 45 degrees.

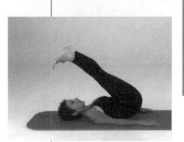

Inhale. Point your toes, bring your legs together and raise them to 90 degrees, ready to begin again.

[5 reps]

Reverse with your legs open and feet flexed on the way up and squeezing them together with pointed toes on the way down.

[5 reps]

SINGLE LEG STRETCH
To strengthen abdominals and improve coordination

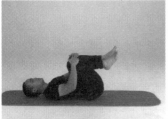

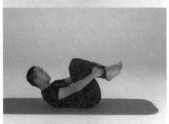

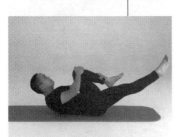

Lie on the mat with a neutral back, knees bent, hands on knees.

Inhale. Lift your head and shoulders off the mat. Keep your ribs anchored.

Slip your hands down your shins towards ankles.

Exhale. As you stretch your right leg away, place right hand on left knee and pull it towards your chest.

Inhale. Bring your knee back and place right hand back on right ankle.

Exhale. Switch your left hand to right knee as left leg stretches away.

Stretch your leg on each exhalation, and come back in on each inhalation.

Keep pace slow, controlled, and constant.

[10 reps]

SINGLE LEG STRETCH WITH ROTATION

To challenge the abdominals and the internal obliques

Lie on your back, knees bent, hands at forehead.

Inhale. Raise your head and shoulders off the mat.

Exhale. Extend left leg to the front and take left elbow to right knee.

Think of a crisscross motion.

Inhale as you extend right leg to the front and take right elbow to left knee.

[10 reps]

Exhale. Relax.

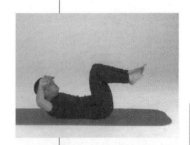

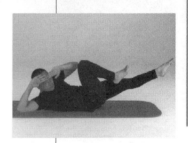

Watchpoints

Keep elbows wide.

Rotate across sternum.

Don't let ribs lighten and lift off mat.

79

DOUBLE LEG STRETCH
To challenge the abdominals and the obliques

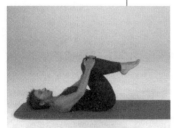

Lie on your back, holding your knees.

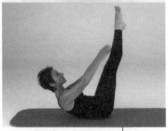

Inhale. Stretch your legs simultaneously with shoulders and head coming off the mat and arms stretched forward in line with the shoulders.

Exhale. Circle your arms backwards overhead while laterally rotating your legs at the hips and flexing your feet (squeeze your thighs together).

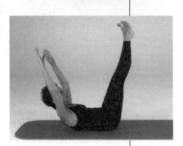

Watchpoint
Be careful not to lower your shoulders towards the mat.

Inhale. Reach upwards to your extended and pointed feet.

Exhale. Place your hands back on bent knees and roll down, bone by bone.

[10 reps]

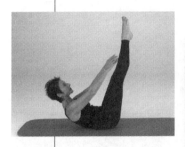

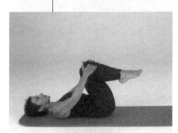

Scissors

To challenge the abdominals and the obliques and further challenge your core stability as you switch legs

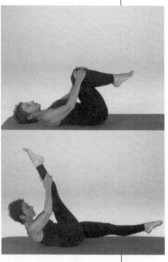

Lie on your back, knees bent, hands on knees.

Inhale. Lift your head and shoulders off the mat, extending one leg horizontally and reaching one leg upwards.

Take hold of the upper leg underneath the calf.

Exhale. Swap legs in mid-air and take hold of the upper leg, pulling it gently towards your trunk and stretching the other leg down.

[20 reps]

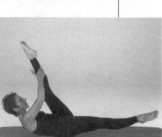

Watchpoint

Don't destabilize the trunk — it should remain anchored on the mat.

Double Leg Kick

To work the back of your legs and buttocks

This exercise also stretches the quadriceps, while giving a gentle stretch to your upper back and across the shoulders.

Lie face down, your legs slightly apart. Interlace your hands, palms up, behind the small of your back. Elbows should be soft and resting on the mat.

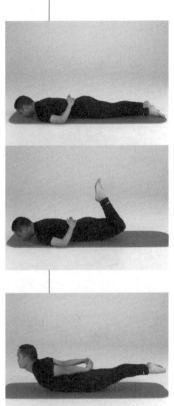

Bend your knees, lifting them slightly off the mat, and flick your heels towards your buttocks three times with three pulses.

Inhale. Release your legs and stretch them out, raising your shoulders to create a stretch across the chest, while your hands turn palm inwards and reach away down your buttocks toward your feet.

Lie down again and repeat the pulses followed by the stretch on the inhalation.

[10 reps]

SIDIES (WAIST TONER)
To strengthen the abdominals, particularly the waist muscles

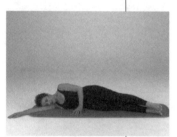

Lie on your right side with hips stacked on top of each other and your head on your outstretched arm.

Use your left hand to gently support your body against the mat – preventing the body from rolling. (I like to think of this hand providing moral rather than actual support.) Your back should be in neutral and your legs in line, toes pointing. However, if you feel your pelvis tilting forward, thereby taking your spine out of neutral, angle your legs slightly forward at the hips.

Inhale. Lengthen your spine parallel to the mat.

Exhale. Lift the muscles at your waist off the mat, then lift legs and trunk simultaneously so that your body is in a line.

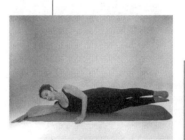

Keep lengthening through your spine and along the back of your neck (the head should float on a continuum with the spine). Feel the muscles at the waist working.

Inhale. Lower the body back and feel the waist muscles imprint the mat.

Exhale. Relax.

Alternate.

[10 reps each side]

When you are confident with the above, allow your upper arm to rest along the side of your body and slide your hand down the side of your thigh as your body lifts. Now let your eyes follow that hand.

[10 reps each side]

Watchpoints

Initiate at the waist. Keep your shoulders down and shoulder blades pulled down the back. Keep eyes focused to the front — back must be neutral.

SIDE KICK

To challenge core stability and increase strength and mobility in hip joint

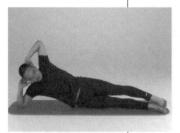

Lie on your left side propped up on your elbow. Support your head with your right hand. Keep your head aligned with your spine.

Place your left hand at the back of your head. Keep elbows out to the side. Position your legs on top of one another in parallel, keeping the hipbones vertically stacked. Angle your legs slightly in front of your body so that your spine can remain neutral.

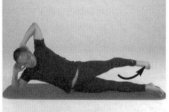
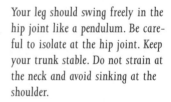

Inhale. Take the left leg to the back with a pointed foot and straight knee.

Exhale. Swing your leg forward with your foot flexed.

Your leg should swing freely in the hip joint like a pendulum. Be careful to isolate at the hip joint. Keep your trunk stable. Do not strain at the neck and avoid sinking at the shoulder.

[10 reps]

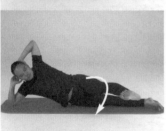

Roll over.

[10 reps]

INSIDE THIGH TONING EXERCISE

To strengthen and tone the adductor muscles of the leg

Lie on your side, ear on your arm, the underneath palm facing the ground, the other hand in front of you gently supporting the body. Place your upper leg over a couple of pillows and bend your knee.

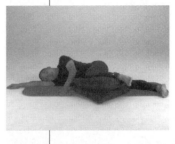

The bottom leg is straight and angled slightly forward at the hip flexor so as to keep the back in neutral.

Inhale.

Exhale. Lift the bottom leg up with flexed foot and bring it down to the mat on the inhale.

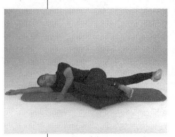

> Be careful to keep the working leg parallel to the mat.

[20 reps]

Now turn over to the other side.

[20 reps]

Watchpoints

This exercise is facilitated by recruiting the abdominals.

You must use the inside thigh to lift the bottom leg.

LEG CIRCLES

To develop core strength, strengthen deep abdominals, and mobilize hip rotator muscles

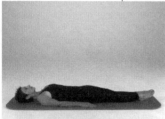

Lie on your back with straight legs.

Inhale. Raise right leg to the ceiling, toes pointed, arms resting by your side.

Exhale. Circle your leg across the left leg.

Inhale as your leg comes back up.

[5 reps]

Exhale and lower leg down to mat.

[5 reps with the left leg]

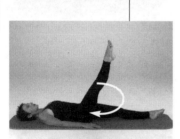

Then circle the other way, with the right leg going away from the left leg.

[Rep 5 times, then rep 5 times with the left leg going away from the right leg]

CAUTION

Keep pelvis in neutral and anchored.

Don't allow buttocks to lift off mat.

ROLLING LIKE A BALL
To massage the spine and strengthen abdominals

Sit on the mat with your legs bent.

Take hold of one wrist and wrap your arms around your legs. Keep your head softly bent forward and gaze down at your navel.

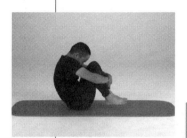

Take your weight slightly behind your tailbone.

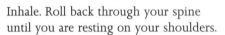

The rounder you are, the better it is.

Inhale. Roll back through your spine until you are resting on your shoulders.

Exhale. Roll back up to a sitting position but do not place your feet on the mat. Use your abdominals to bring you back upright.

[10 reps]

CAUTION

Do not do this exercise if you have osteoporosis, a back problem, or any discomfort in the spine.

THE HUNDRED

To increase core stability by improving muscle control, enhancing breathing capacity, and reoxygenating and pumping blood around the body

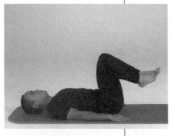

Lie on your back, knees bent, feet parallel, arms by your sides, palms facing down.

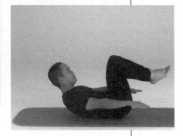

Inhale. Raise knees, head, and shoulders.

Exhale. Extend both legs out to 90 degrees. Lower them a little towards the mat, if you can't keep your back in neutral.

Using your arms as a pump and keeping time with your breathing, breathe out 5 times and in 5 times.

Keep your elbows straight and arms strong.

[10 reps — until you have completed a hundred beats]

Inhale. Bring your knees to bent position.

Exhale. Roll back to the mat.

Remember to keep a neutral spine.

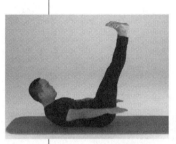

If this is too intense, the Hundred can be done with knees bent and thighs vertical, thus shortening the levers you have to hold up. Or you can keep both feet on the mat.

Spine Stretch

To stretch the spine, stretch hamstrings (although the emphasis is on the spine), and stabilize the trunk

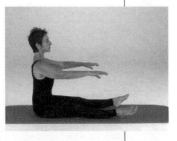

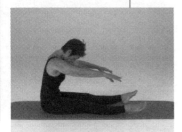

Sit tall on your sitting bones with your legs apart at a comfortable distance. (Your knees may remain bent if you feel the impulse to roll back off your tailbone and compromise your upright position.)

Keep your toes soft. Keep arms at shoulder height and parallel to legs. Lift up out of the hips and imagine that your back is supported by a wall.

Inhale. Peel off and flex cervical (upper) spine.

Drop your chin forward and curl down toward your crotch.

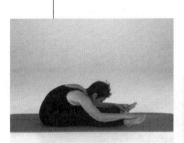

Exhale. Feel your head stretch along parallel to your legs and place your hands under the balls of your feet, lengthening and stretching the spine.

Inhale. Return your spine to the intermediate position (cervical flexion).

Exhale. Restack your spine bone by bone until the spine is rebuilt and your head is upright.

[6 reps]

Watchpoints

Keep your shoulder blades in their stabilized position and your neck long and free.

Breathe into your backbone.

THE SAW

To stretch spine, sides, inner thighs, and ham-strings, and to stabilize center

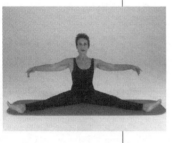

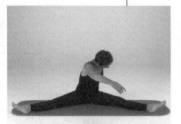

Sit up tall on your sitting bones.

Stretch your legs in a wide V shape. Keep your toes soft.

Lift out of the hips and length-en spine. Open your arms to your sides. Slide your shoulder blades down your back.

Inhale. Rotate your body to the left and take your upper cervical spine into flexion. You are fac-ing your left leg.

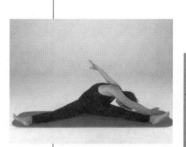

With 3 pulsing exhalations, reach forward and down so that the back of your right hand slides down the outside of your left foot with 3 sawing movements.

Reach your hand further on each pulse. Do not jerk.

Inhale. Roll spine back to intermediate position, still facing the right leg.

Exhale. Bring the body back to the center and restack the spine.

Repeat on the other side.

[10 reps each side]

Watchpoints

Don't roll the thigh of the opposite leg.

Keep buttocks on the mat.

Slide shoulder blades down your back.

SPINE TWIST

To improve the mobility of the thorax, stretch the spine, and wring the bad air from the lungs

Watchpoints

Do not sink into your pelvic girdle.

Lift tall out of your waist.

Lengthen your neck and spine by pressing up from the crown of the head.

Make sure you don't force your head past the point of comfort.

Sit up tall on your sitting bones.

Straighten your legs out in front of you, hip-width apart, feet flexed, and heels pressing into the floor.

Stretch your arms out to either side

Inhale. Zip up, hollow and scoop, from the navel.

Exhale. Twist your trunk to the right. Keep pulling up out of the hips. Add a pulse to release the air out of your lungs.

Imagine you are wringing water from a wet towel.

Inhale. Return your trunk to the front. Keep your shoulder blades down and your arms outstretched.

Exhale. Repeat the twist to the left.

Inhale. Return your trunk to the front.

[10 reps each side]

Exhale to relax.

THE PLANK

To strengthen the back muscles as well as developing cross-diagonal support and to challenge the arms, shoulder girdle, and abdominals

Kneel on all fours and place forearms on the mat with hands clasped. Raise yourself up onto the balls of your feet like a jack-knife and walk them away from your center until your body forms a straight line between shoulders and tailbone.

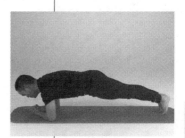

Hold for as long as you can maintain your form.

To increase the challenge, do the Plank with straight arms, keeping your hands directly under shoulders and elbows straight.

Watchpoints

Keep your legs straight, and your shoulder blades pulled down and stabilized.

Most importantly, abdominals contract to support the spine.

PUSH-UPS

To strengthen shoulders, chest, arms, upper back, and abdominals

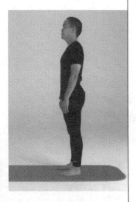

This exercise is an alternative to the Plank.

Stand straight with legs and feet parallel, arms by your side, abdominals drawn in towards your backbone.

Inhale.

Exhale. Lower your hands down the front of your legs and place palms flat on the mat. You will feel a hamstring stretch.

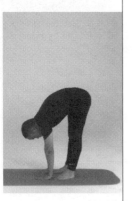

Inhale. Walk your hands away until they are directly under your shoulders.

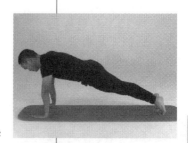

Exhale. Bring your hips down until they are in line with the rest of your body. Make a line from the tip of your head to the back of your heels.

Inhale. Bend your elbows. Try to keep them close to your ribs. Make certain that your abdominals remain engaged.

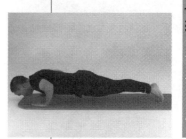

Exhale. Push up, straightening your elbows.

[6 reps]

Stay down on the last push-up with elbows bent and hold for 6 seconds, breathing normally.

Inhale. Stretch your elbows and walk hands back to feet. Try to keep your knees straight.

Exhale. Roll your body back to upright position.

[3 reps]

CORKSCREW *A
To strengthen and challenge core muscles

This can only be done if you can fully straighten your knees.

Lie on your back in constructive rest with your arms on the mat beside you.

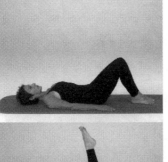

Inhale. Unfold your legs so that they are perpendicular to your hips.

Point your toes and make sure that your knees are straight.

Exhale. Circle legs clockwise.

Inhale. Reverse cycle.

[10 reps]

Inhale. Bend your knees.

Exhale. Stretch your legs back onto the mat.

Watchpoints

The circles should be small.

The pelvis should be anchored — steady and square.

The tailbone stays down.

Roll Down the Wall

To develop coordination of the upper body, learn how to wheel the spine bone by bone, and achieve synchronous segmental control using the stabilizers

Stand with your back against the wall with your feet approx 12" (45 cm) away.

Your shoulder blades and seat should touch the wall but the back of the head and the middle back do not. Dangle your arms.

Bend knees, feet hip-width apart, weight evenly balanced.

> Think of the xiphoid process as the fulcrum of the roll down.

Inhale.

Exhale. Drop your chin to your chest and let the weight of your head begin the process. Peel your bones off the wall, bone by bone, arms dangling vertically from shoulders. Breathe in as you hang forward, like a rag doll.

Exhale. Drop your tailbone down, directing your pubic bone forward. Hollow the abdominals, rotate the pelvis backwards as you slowly roll the bones back onto the wall, one by one until you are back to your starting position.

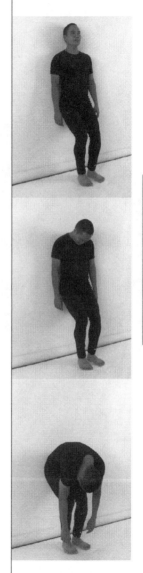

LARGE HIP ROLLS

To mobilize the spine and stretch lower back and hips

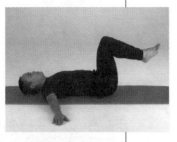

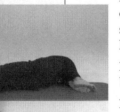

Lie on your back, with your arms stretched out to the side, palms facing down and below shoulder level. Raise your legs with knees bent, thighs at 90 degrees.

Inhale.

Exhale. Treating the two legs as one unit, roll them over to one side of the body and rotate your head in the opposite direction.

Inhale. Bring your legs and head back to the center.

Exhale. Roll your bent knees in the other direction. Turn your head to the opposite side.

[10 reps]

Rest Position

To stretch out lumbar, middle, and upper spine

Position yourself on all fours.

Bring your feet together. If you want to feel a stretch in your inner thighs, keep your knees apart. If your knees are together, the emphasis will be on a lumbar stretch.

Move your body back onto your buttocks and sit on your feet. Keep your back rounded and place your face down on the mat, arms extended to give you the maximum stretch.

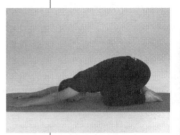

Inhale. Feel your rib cage and back expand.

Exhale. Recruit your abdominals and think of dropping your tailbone down.

[Repeat for 10 breaths]

CAUTION

Avoid this stretch if you have knee problems.

On the Go

Short Powerhouse Workout & the Tall Diamond,
Medium Workout, Long Workout

THE SHORT POWERHOUSE WORKOUT

- *To integrate the mind and body*
- *To integrate the trunk with the upper and lower structures of the body*
- *To develop core strength*
- *To develop an awareness of the relationship between the pelvis and lower back*
- *To develop an awareness of the deep abdominals*

If you are pushed for time, just fall out of bed, do this 15-minute workout and you'll be set for the day.

1. Anchoring the Trunk

Lie on your back, knees in constructive rest, feet hip-width apart, arms resting at your side. Alternatively, raise your legs with thighs vertical and knees bent as shown.

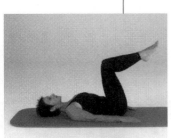

Inhale through your nose. Feel your breath fill the back and expand your ribs laterally.

Exhale through your mouth. Feel your lower abdomen draw in toward the mat and up toward your navel, narrowing at the waist. The ribs should soften down and narrow, decreasing the distance between the ribs and pelvis.

Imagine your breathing as the ebb and flow of waves.

[10 reps]

2. Integrating the Arm & Trunk
To stretch the latissimus dorsi muscles

Lift your arms, holding them vertical in line with your shoulders.

Keep shoulders wide and don't let your arms come in toward your ears. Raise legs with knees bent, thighs vertical.

Inhale.

Exhale. Lower your arms behind you.

Inhale. Keep pelvis stable, return arms to vertical.

[10 reps]

Exhale.

Watchpoints

Be very careful not to let any part of your trunk lift off the mat as you reach away from the center. You may not be able to place your arms on the mat if your latissimus dorsi muscles are tight. You should feel comfortable with the movement.

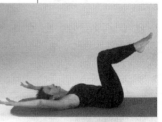

3. Coordinating the Limbs & Anchoring the Trunk

- *To strengthen the abdominals*
- *To improve coordination*

Remain lying with your legs raised and bent and your arms vertical.

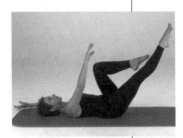

Inhale.

Exhale. Extend your right arm back overhead and left leg away from body (at about 45 degrees).

The further you lengthen the arm and leg away from your trunk, the harder it is to keep the abdominal connection.

Inhale. Return both limbs to the starting position.

Alternate legs and arms.

[10 reps]

Exhale.

4. Double Arm & Leg Stretch *A
To further challenge the abdominals

Remain lying with legs bent and arms vertical.

Inhale.

Exhale. Carefully stretch arms and legs away from your center.

> Treat this movement as an abdominal teaser. It is not essential to fully stretch your limbs away, but make sure that the trunk remains anchored.

Inhale. Return your limbs to the starting position.

[10 reps]

Exhale.

This stretch is a little more challenging and should only be done if your abdominals are strong enough. Otherwise the effort may transfer into your back.

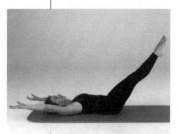

On the Go Short Workout

5. The Clam

- *To work adductors*
- *To work lateral hip rotators*
- *To improve coordination*
- *To develop awareness of centering*

Remain lying with legs bent and arms vertical.

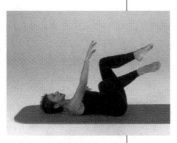

Inhale.

Exhale. Open your right knee to the side while simultaneously opening the opposite arm to the other side.

Inhale. Bring your limbs back to the starting position.

[10 reps, alternating sides]

Exhale. Relax.

THE TALL DIAMOND

To exercise all the abdominals for ultimate core strength

This exercise is an alternative to the Short Powerhouse Workout.

Step 1.

Lie on your back with your hands at the back of your head. Keep your elbows out to the side. Extend your legs directly above your hips and form a tall diamond shape by bending your knees at an obtuse angle and crossing your ankles.

Inhale.

Halfway through the exhalation, bring your head and shoulders off the mat and hold for the remainder of the exhalation (approximately 3 seconds).

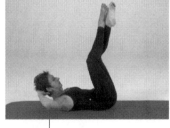

Try to articulate the bones of the upper back as they roll off the mat by keeping your ribcage anchored as much as possible. Use your xiphoid process as the fulcrum.

Inhale. Roll the head and shoulders back to the mat.

[10 reps with one ankle in front]

Exhale and rest.

[10 reps with other ankle in front]

Step 2.

Position your body as for Step 1.

Inhale.

Exhale. Halfway through the exhalation, bring your head and shoulders off the mat and rotate to one side, using the elbow that you are turning towards as a pivot. Rotate your shoulders and do not let your ribs lift off the mat. Hold for a further 3 seconds, continuing to exhale.

Inhale. Roll back down to the mat.

Exhale.

[5 reps, rotating to the same side]

Switch ankles.

[5 reps, rotating to the other side]

Exhale and rest.

[Repeat Step 2]

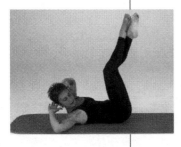

Watchpoints

Keep your ribs anchored.

Only rotate across the chest.

Sample Medium Workout

Warm Up/Stretches

Quad Stretch (page 39)

Chest Stretch (page 62)

Hamstring Stretch (page 60)

Side Stretch (page 57)

Workout

Turtle (page 63)

Abdominal Preparation or
Roll-Up (page 70, 72 & 74)

Single Leg Stretch with
Rotation (page 79)

Cat (page 67)

Medium Workout (cont.)

Single Leg Stretch (page 78)

Large Hip Roll (page 102)

Sidies (page 84)

Spine Stretch (page 92)

Leg Circles (page 88)

Push-Ups (page 98)

The Hundred (page 90)

Sample Long Workout

Warm Up/Stretches

Arm Opening (page 51)

Hip Flexor Stretch (page 58)

Basic Wall Stretch I (page 52)

Basic Wall Stretch II (page 53)

Workout

Sergeant Major (Dart)
(page 66)

Roll-Up (page 72)

Single Leg Stretch (page 78)

Double Leg Stretch (page 80)

On the Go Long Workout

Long Workout (cont.)

Pelvic Press (page 69)

Side Kick (page 86)

Single Leg Stretch with
Rotation (page 79)

Scissors (page 82)

Double Leg Kick (page 83)

Rolling Like a Ball (page 89)

The Saw & Spine Twist
(page 94–6)

The Hundred (page 90)

Long Workout (cont.)

Leg Circles (page 88)

Spine Stretch (page 92)

The Plank (page 97)

Roll Down the Wall
(page 101)

Glossary

biceps: Muscles on the inside of the arm that originate at the elbow and insert at the armpit.

constructive rest: Position on the back, knees comfortably bent, feet parallel on floor, hip-width apart, toes in the same line as legs. The back is in neutral with relaxed neck, shoulders, and head.

core stability: In Pilates the core muscles are called the powerhouse. This constitutes the group of muscles from the diaphragm to the pelvic floor, including the abdominal muscles, buttock muscles, lower back muscles and the whole pelvic function. The abdominal muscles surround and support the lower trunk and connect the pelvis to the ribs. The six-pack or rectus abdominus is the flavor of the month, but in fact it is the most superficial of all the abdominals. Pilates is much more preoccupied with the deeper stabilizing abdominals, which act as our second spine – they are the external and internal obliques that wrap themselves around the waist. The internal obliques help bend and spirally twist the trunk as well as flattening the stomach. The external obliques help with side bending, twisting and rotation of the trunk, and narrowing of the waist. The muscles of the transversus abdominis form the deepest layer and provide support to the internal organs. When contracted it pulls the abdominal wall toward the spine. The four abdominal muscles form a corset from the pubic bone to the ribs and wrap around the body right to the spine. It is only when you are breathing correctly that you can activate the correct lateral and deep abdominal muscles.

DVT: Deep Vein Thrombosis.

erector spinae: Thick muscles oriented vertically along the longitudinal axis of the back.

glutei: Buttock muscles that are arranged in three layers: gluteus maximus, gluteus medius, gluteus minimus.

hamstrings: Muscles & tendons that run up the back of the leg from the knee to the buttocks.

iliopsoas: Three hip flexors that are referred to in combination with one another as the iliopsoas. The iliopsoas also flexes the lumbar vertebrae.

Jin Shin Jyutsu: An ancient Japanese therapy that reduces stress and pain, and balances emotions.

lumbar spine: Five vertebrae in the vertebral column that are massive weight-bearing bones with limited mobility.

metatarsal: Five long bones in the foot.

neutral: The correct natural shape of the spine and pelvis. If the top of the pelvis tips forward, the lumbar curve increases. If it tips back, the lumbar spine flattens. Neutral is the position between the two extremes.

oblique muscles: External oblique muscles are deep abdominal muscles that run on either side of the vertical front muscles called the rectus abdominis. Below these, at the side, are the internal obliques.

pelvic floor: This is made up of the urethra and vagina or penis and testes in front, and the anus at the back, surrounded by a band of muscle called the perineum.

the Powerhouse: The band of muscles that encircles the body, extending from the lower ribcage to the pelvic floor.

pulses: Short shallow movements made in time with short shallow exhalations.

quadriceps: Muscles that run along the front of the thigh originating at the knee and inserting at the hip.

recruit: To engage a specific group of muscles.

rectus abdominis: Vertical abdominal muscle running from the pubic bone to the sternum. It is located superficially.

sacrum: Five fused bones at the base of the vertebral column.

Thera-Band™: A long piece of elasticised rubber.

thoracic: The twelve thoracic vertebrae of the vertebral column articulate with the ribs.

transversus abdominis: Muscles that wrap around the abdomen in the deepest layer.

triceps: Muscles that originate at the elbow and insert at the armpit.

wheeling: Articulating the spinal column bone by bone while engaging the abdominals at the front.

xiphoid process: A small projection at the base of the sternum.

zip up, hollow and scoop: The process of drawing the transversus abdominis and pelvic floor inward and upward to create a concave appearance in the belly and a narrowing of the waist.

Index